Compete and Comply:

How Narcissists Use Triangulation to Manipulate Their Supply

Jacquette Brown, MS, LPC-S

Legal Disclaimer

This book is for informational purposes only and is not a substitute for professional medical, psychological, or legal advice. The author and publisher are not liable for any outcomes resulting from its use. If you experience distress or a mental health crisis, please seek support from a qualified professional or contact a crisis helpline. In the U.S., you can reach the National Suicide Prevention Lifeline at 988 or visit 988lifeline.org for confidential support 24/7.

Table of Contents

Acknowledgments...1

About the author's bio 2

Introduction 3

Chapter 1: What Is Triangulation?...6

Chapter 2: The Narcissistic Supply Chain 13

Chapter 3: The Three Roles in Triangulation........................21

Chapter 4: Romantic Triangulation..27

Chapter 5: Familial Triangulation..33

Chapter 6: Workplace Triangulation......................................38

Chapter 7: Social and Friendship Circles...............................45

Chapter 8: Recognizing When You're Being Triangulated ...50

Chapter 9: Strategies to Disengage 56

Chapter 10: Healing and Moving Forward 63

Conclusion of All Chapters...69

Interactive Journal: Reflecting on Narcissistic Triangulation
and Healing 73

Acknowledgments

Thank you to my family and friends for your unwavering support and encouragement. To my readers, this book is for you. Self-publishing has been a journey, and I'm grateful for every lesson along the way.

With appreciation,

Jacquette Brown, MS, LPC-S

About the author's bio

Jacquette Brown, MS, LPC-S is a dedicated Licensed Professional Counselor with a passion for unraveling the complexities of the human mind. With a master's degree in Forensic Psychology and Professional Counseling, she specializes in trauma treatment and personality disorders, particularly Cluster B diagnoses. Her deep interest in Narcissistic Personality Disorder (NPD) fuels her work by shedding light on its impact and pathways to healing. As an author, she blends clinical expertise with real-world insights, offering readers a compelling and compassionate perspective on mental health and recovery.

Introduction

Triangulation—the narcissist's favorite pastime. Why settle for one person's admiration when you can have two (or more) fighting for approval? It's the psychological equivalent of dangling a shiny toy just out of reach, watching as people scramble to prove their worth. For the narcissist, it's all about control: Who's in favor today? Who's being iced out? Who needs to try harder? The answer, of course, is everyone—because no amount of effort is ever enough. The result? You're left anxious, second-guessing yourself, and walking on eggshells.

The beauty of triangulation—at least from their perspective—is how effortless it is. A casual mention of an ex, a backhanded compliment, or a whisper of gossip is enough to send others into emotional chaos, while the narcissist sits back, feigning innocence. Whether it's a romantic partner questioning their worth, siblings competing for attention, or coworkers tearing each other down, the narcissist orchestrates the drama and feeds on the fallout.

This is narcissistic abuse: a relentless cycle of being built up, torn down, and strung along with just enough hope to keep you playing their rigged game. The grand prize? Constant self-doubt and the realization that you'll never "win." Every reaction you give—whether scrambling for approval, competing with others, or complying for affection—is their trophy. To keep you hooked, they'll shift the rules, gaslight your reality, and convince you that the problem is you: you're overreacting, too sensitive, or just jealous. Meanwhile, the truth is that you're being manipulated into forgetting who you are.

So why this book? Because it's time to flip the script. Triangulation is a game you never agreed to play, and it's time to stop. Here, we'll pull back the curtain on the narcissist's favorite tactics, expose their strategies, and give you the tools to reclaim your power.

Understand this: triangulation isn't always loud or dramatic. Sometimes it's subtle, almost elegant in its cruelty. A partner casually mentions an ex. A boss praises one colleague while dismissing you with faint praise. A sibling rivalry is quietly stoked. Even friendships can become battlegrounds under the guise of "harmless" comparisons. The common thread? You're left questioning yourself, while the narcissist savors the control.

And yes, it's exhausting—like playing a game you never signed up for. One wrong move and you're the villain, one "right" move and you're still never enough. But here's the truth: You're not crazy. You're not too sensitive. And you don't have to keep proving your worth to someone who thrives on making you feel replaceablc.

Once you recognize the game, the rules lose their power. You don't need to compete, comply, or grovel for affection that isn't real. You don't need to stay in a circus designed to keep you small. Awareness is the turning point—the moment you stop being a pawn and start reclaiming your life.

So pay attention, take notes, and brace yourself. Because once you see triangulation for what it is, you won't just survive the narcissist's twisted game—you'll end it.

Game over.

The Psychology of Triangulation

Chapter 1:
What Is Triangulation?

The Origins of the Term in Psychology

If narcissists had a rulebook, triangulation would be listed as one of their Top 10 favorite manipulation tactics. Why? Because it's simple, effective, and creates the kind of drama that keeps them at the center of everyone's world. They thrive on chaos, so why not create it? Nothing cements their power like watching people fight for their validation, scramble for their attention, or question their own reality—all while the narcissist sits back and enjoys the show. But where did this game come from? Is it just something narcissists instinctively know how to do, or does it have an actual psychological foundation? Turns out, it does. And, as usual, narcissists have taken a legitimate psychological concept and twisted it into a weapon of mass emotional destruction.

The Psychological Foundation: Bowen's Family Systems Theory

Triangulation, as a psychological concept, was first introduced by psychiatrist Dr. Murray Bowen as part of his Family Systems Theory. Bowen observed that when tension arises between two people, a third person is often pulled in to relieve stress or stabilize the situation. In a healthy setting, triangulation can serve as a temporary coping mechanism—like when a child mediates between arguing parents or when a friend helps resolve a misunderstanding between two others. Ideally, this third person helps calm things down, rather than making them worse.

However, Bowen also noted that while a triangle is more stable than a dyad, it creates an "odd person out," which can be a difficult position for individuals to tolerate. Anxiety generated by being or anticipating being the odd person out is a potent force in triangles. This dynamic can complicate relationships and perpetuate unhealthy patterns if not managed properly.

Narcissistic Manipulation: Twisting Triangulation

But here's where things get ugly. While Bowen's triangulation was about reducing stress and restoring balance, narcissists use it for the exact opposite purpose: to create tension, insecurity, and emotional chaos. Instead of using a third party to resolve conflict, they introduce one to manufacture it. In their version of triangulation, they aren't looking to make peace—they're looking to stir the pot and keep everyone hooked on the cycle of competition and compliance.

The reason this works so well is that humans are wired to seek validation and avoid rejection. Narcissists know this, and they exploit it masterfully. By making someone feel like they are in direct competition with another person for the narcissist's approval, they create an emotional storm that leaves their victims desperate, off-balance, and easier to control. It's not just manipulation; it's psychological warfare, and narcissists are disturbingly good at it.

How It Works in Relationships

If you've ever found yourself competing for someone's attention, affection, or approval—and you didn't even sign up for the competition—congratulations, you've been triangulated. This manipulation tactic works in all kinds of relationships: romantic, familial, workplace, and friendships. The only requirement? A narcissist who thrives on control and an unsuspecting victim (or two) who doesn't realize they're being played.

Romantic Relationships: Picture this—you're dating someone, things are going great, and then suddenly, they start casually mentioning their ex. Not in a "Wow, I'm so glad that's over" way, but more like, "They were so amazing at cooking, I'll never find someone like them again." Or maybe they're always texting a "friend" who conveniently seems to pop up whenever you express a need for more attention. The message? *You're not enough. You need to try harder. You can be replaced.* And just like that, you're working overtime to prove your worth to someone who *never intended to appreciate you in the first place.*

Familial Relationships: The classic *Golden Child vs. Scapegoat* dynamic. Narcissistic parents are experts at pitting their children against each other. One day, you're the shining star, the next, you're the disappointment. Meanwhile, your sibling is going through the exact same thing—just in reverse. The parent's goal? Keep their children competing for love, ensuring that neither ever feels secure enough to question the system. It's a masterclass in emotional control, and unfortunately, it can leave deep psychological scars long into adulthood.

Workplace Drama: Have a boss who seems to play favorites? One minute, you're the go-to employee, the next, you're getting the cold shoulder while someone else basks in their praise. Narcissistic managers love to create workplace competition because it keeps employees too distracted fighting for their approval to ever notice that they're being exploited. If you've ever worked in an environment where coworkers were pitted against each other rather than encouraged to collaborate, you've witnessed workplace triangulation in action.

Friendships and Social Circles: Ever had a friend who made sure you *knew* they had other, *better* friends? Maybe they drop little comments about how much fun they had with someone else, or maybe they make a habit of excluding you just enough to keep you on edge. The goal? To keep you vying for their attention, always feeling like you need to "prove" that you're worthy of their time. It's not friendship; it's a game, and the narcissist is the only one who ever wins.

Why Narcissists Use Triangulation as a Control Tactic

Now, the big question: Why? Why go through the trouble of manipulating people into competing for them? Wouldn't it be easier to just form normal, healthy relationships? *Sure, but where's the fun in that?*

Triangulation serves a few key purposes for a narcissist:

1. **It Keeps You Insecure and Dependent.** When you never feel "good enough," you work harder to please them. The more you seek their approval, the more power they have over you. It's a never-ending cycle that keeps you locked into their world.

2. **It Creates Drama (Which They Love).** Narcissists thrive on emotional chaos. Watching people scramble for their affection gives them an ego boost. It reassures them that they are *important enough* to have people fighting over them.

3. **It Distracts You from Their Toxicity.** When you're too busy proving yourself, you don't have time to notice that the real problem is *them*. If you're too wrapped up in jealousy, competition, or confusion, you won't call them out on their behavior.

4. **It Makes You More Tolerant of Their Abuse.** If they make you feel like you *could* be replaced, you're more likely to tolerate mistreatment. You'll excuse their bad behavior, overlook the red flags, and settle for whatever breadcrumbs of affection they choose to throw your way.

At its core, triangulation is all about power. The narcissist creates an illusion of scarcity—whether it's love, attention, or approval—and convinces you that you must fight for it. The truth? There is no competition. There never was. The game is rigged from the start, designed to keep *you* in a state of self-doubt and *them* in complete control.

But here's where things change. The moment you see triangulation for what it is, you take away its power. The narcissist's greatest weapon is confusion, and clarity is their greatest threat. The second you recognize the manipulation, you can step out of the cycle. And trust me—nothing terrifies a narcissist more than someone who stops playing their game.

Chapter 2:
The Narcissistic Supply Chain

If narcissists were cars, they wouldn't run on gas—they'd run on attention, admiration, and the sweet, sweet sound of people desperately trying to please them. This is what's known as *narcissistic supply*, the lifeblood that keeps them going. Without a steady dose of praise, validation, and emotional turmoil to feed on, a narcissist is about as useful as a phone with 1% battery—desperate, irrational, and frantically searching for a charger (aka their next victim).

Of course, a single source of supply is never enough. Oh no, narcissists need *options*. They build an entire network—like an emotional Ponzi scheme—where different people provide different types of validation at all times. Some are there to worship them, others to fight for their approval, and a select few to be torn down just for sport. Because what's the point of being a puppet master if you don't have enough puppets?

Understanding Narcissistic Supply

Narcissistic supply is exactly what it sounds like—a never-ending stream of emotional resources that keep a narcissist functioning. But let's be clear: this isn't about love, connection, or mutual respect. No, narcissists don't crave *relationships*; they crave *control*. They don't want companionship; they want compliance. And they don't need you as a person—they need you as a mirror, constantly reflecting back the image they want to see.

Think of it like an addiction. Normal people find fulfillment in genuine human connection, but narcissists? They're junkies for attention. The highs come from admiration, flattery, and being the center of the universe. The lows? Well, that's when they need drama, chaos, and someone to emotionally bleed out in front of them so they can feel superior. Either way, it's all supply. Whether they're basking in praise or relishing someone's emotional breakdown, as long as they are *the reason* for someone's intense emotional state, they're winning.

And, like any good addict, a narcissist will do whatever it takes to get their fix. If compliments aren't rolling in fast enough, they'll throw a pity party and soak up sympathy. If admiration runs low, they'll manufacture jealousy or insecurity to stir the pot. If attention wanes, they'll start a fight just to make sure *someone* is thinking about them. To a narcissist, emotional energy—good or bad—is the currency that keeps their world spinning. And trust me, they are *always* collecting.

Primary vs. Secondary Supply

Now, not all supply sources are created equal. There's a hierarchy, a carefully crafted system where different people serve different roles. Welcome to the twisted world of *Primary vs. Secondary Supply*, where narcissists assign people value based on how much control they can exert over them.

> **Primary Supply:** This is the VIP section. The crème de la crème of validation. Primary supply is usually a romantic partner, a devoted best friend, or a family member who has been sufficiently conditioned to revolve their entire existence around the narcissist's needs. These poor souls provide the *deepest* levels of supply—unwavering admiration, unconditional emotional energy, and, ideally, complete self-sacrifice. They're expected to *worship* the narcissist, soothe their insecurities, and, most importantly, never, ever outshine them. Because the second they stop feeding the narcissist's ego, they become expendable.

> **Secondary Supply:** Yes, the backup dancers in the narcissist's never-ending performance. Secondary supply consists of acquaintances, coworkers, social media followers, and even exes kept on emotional life support just in case the

primary source starts slacking. These people provide surface-level attention—likes, compliments, a little harmless flirting, or the occasional "You're so amazing" text. They might not be fully locked into the narcissist's gravitational pull, but their presence still serves a purpose. After all, a narcissist needs a constant rotation of admiration to keep the illusion alive.

The genius of this system? If the primary supply starts getting a little *too* independent (or worse, starts realizing they deserve better), the narcissist simply leans on their secondary supply. It's like having multiple credit cards—when one gets maxed out, they just switch to another. And because they've spent a lifetime perfecting this juggling act, they always make sure they have *just enough* emotional investors to keep their empire running.

Why Narcissists Keep Multiple Sources of Supply

At this point, you might be wondering, *Wouldn't it just be easier to have one stable, devoted partner instead of an entire supply chain?* You'd think, right? But for a narcissist, stability is boring, commitment is restrictive, and having only one person to manipulate is too much pressure. They don't just want supply—they want variety. They want multiple sources of admiration, attention, and emotional energy so that if one begins to run dry, another is ready and waiting.

It's not about love or connection—it's about maintaining a constant feedback loop that reassures them of their superiority and control. One person can't supply enough fuel for a narcissist's ego; they need a rotation of people to compare, compete, and comply, all under their influence. Think of it like a gourmet buffet, except instead of food, it's attention, adoration, and emotional energy.

And here's where it gets truly insidious: they create subtle drama among their supply individually, behind the scenes. While each person believes they are the "favorite" or most trusted, the narcissist quietly smears the others behind the scenes, planting doubts and whispering half-truths to fuel insecurity and competition, keeping everyone either at a distance or at odds.

One partner might hear an offhand comment implying another is jealous or untrustworthy, while a coworker receives a casual remark painting someone else as incompetent or unreliable. No one ever sees the whole picture, but everyone feels the tension and starts scrambling to secure their position.

By doing this, the narcissist ensures that each person remains off-balance, questioning themselves and the intentions of others, all while the narcissist maintains a smug sense of omnipotence. Each supply becomes both a pawn and a competitor, creating a perfect cycle of anxiety, overcompensation, and dependence. Stability would be too simple; they thrive on manipulation, subtle chaos, and the illusion that they are always in control.

Variety allows them to test boundaries, sow confusion, and keep each person vying for their approval without ever committing fully to any single one. One partner might be praised for a minor achievement while another is quietly undermined, and all of it happens with such subtlety that it often goes unnoticed until the damage is done. For the narcissist, this behind-the-scenes drama is just as thrilling as the public adoration—they feed off the tension, competition, and compliance like it's a carefully crafted art form.

So yes, a devoted partner might sound convenient—but for a narcissist, convenience is deadly boring. They need the drama, the unpredictability, and the constant flow of validation from multiple angles. One partner might be enough for love, but never enough for control. And control? That's the true currency of their world.

Having multiple sources of supply serves several key (and completely self-serving) purposes:

1. **It Keeps Everyone on Edge.** Nothing fuels a narcissist's power trip like knowing people are

competing for them. If one source of supply starts getting too comfortable, they'll subtly (or not so subtly) remind them that there are *others*. Maybe it's casually bringing up an ex, gushing over a coworker, or making sure their social media is filled with admiration from admirers. The message is clear: *You are replaceable. Keep performing.*

2. **It Provides a Safety Net.** Narcissists know that people eventually get tired of their nonsense. So, like a paranoid doomsday prepper stockpiling canned goods, they make sure they have *backup supply* ready to go. If their primary source starts pulling away, they can immediately redirect their energy to someone else—because God forbid they sit with their own thoughts for five minutes.

3. **It Feeds Their Ego From Every Angle.** One person telling them they're amazing is nice, but a *horde* of admirers? That's the dream. Whether it's romantic partners, friends, colleagues, or social media followers, narcissists thrive on a *constant* stream of validation. The more people singing their praises, the more powerful they feel.

4. **It Shields Them From Accountability.** If one person calls them out on their toxic behavior, they just hop over to another supply source for

reassurance. "My partner thinks I'm manipulative? Time to call my ex and hear about how much they still miss me." "My coworker thinks I take credit for their work? No problem, my boss thinks I'm a genius." There's always another person ready to stroke their ego, so they never have to *actually* reflect on their actions.

At the end of the day, narcissists keep multiple sources of supply because *they have to*. Their entire sense of self is propped up by external validation, and without it, they start crumbling. Unlike emotionally healthy people, who can find self-worth within themselves, narcissists are *entirely* dependent on outside admiration. And the second that admiration disappears? So does their illusion of superiority.

But here's the thing—once you understand how the supply chain works, you stop being part of it. The minute you recognize that you're not *special* to a narcissist (just another cog in their validation machine), you gain the power to step off the ride. And nothing terrifies a narcissist more than losing their supply.

So, the real question is: Are you going to keep playing your assigned role, or are you ready to shut down their supply chain for good?

Chapter 3:
The Three Roles in Triangulation

If narcissists had a favorite hobby—besides self-worship—it would be *triangulation*. There's nothing they love more than setting people up against each other, sitting back, and enjoying the emotional gladiator match they orchestrated. To pull off this masterpiece of manipulation, they assign *roles*. And no, you don't get to pick yours. That would imply you have control, and we can't have that now, can we?

Triangulation operates like a never-ending, badly written soap opera where the narcissist is both the director and the main character. The rest of you? You're just playing your part—whether you like it or not. Today, you might be the beloved *Favored Supply*, but don't get comfortable. Tomorrow, you could be the *Devalued Supply*. And through it all, there's one person who never loses: *the narcissist, the Puppet Master in Chief.*

The Favored Supply (Golden Child, Idealized Partner, Best Employee)

The *Chosen One*! This is the role that everyone *thinks* they want—until they realize it comes with more strings attached than a marionette doll. The Favored Supply is the narcissist's prized possession, showered with compliments, love-bombed into oblivion, and paraded around like a trophy. Whether it's the *Golden Child* in a narcissistic family, the *Idealized Partner* in a relationship, or the *Best Employee* at work, this person is temporarily the apple of the narcissist's eye.

> **Golden Child:** In a narcissistic family, the Golden Child is placed on a pedestal so high that they're practically oxygen-deprived. They are the "perfect" kid, the one who "makes the family proud." But make no mistake—this isn't unconditional love. This is *conditional worship*. The moment the Golden Child stops making the narcissistic parent look good, they'll be knocked off that pedestal so fast their head will spin.

> **Idealized Partner:** Romantic partners in the idealization phase are treated like royalty—until they aren't. In the beginning, they are "the best thing that's ever happened" to the narcissist. Compliments flow, grand gestures are made, and

they are told they are *different* from everyone else. The catch? The second they stop being *perfect*, the narcissist begins their slow descent into the next role: the Devalued Supply.

Best Employee: At work, the narcissist's Favorite Employee is praised endlessly—until they become a threat. They might be given extra responsibilities, trusted with projects, and told they are the "most valuable team member." But the second they outshine the narcissistic boss, or (worse) start expecting fair treatment, their days in the spotlight are numbered.

The trickiest part of being the Favored Supply? It feels *so good* at first. The love, the praise, the validation—it's intoxicating. But the reality is that it's *never* about you. It's about how well you serve the narcissist's ego. And the moment you stop feeding their need for control? You'll be tossed aside faster than last year's trending influencer.

The Devalued Supply (Scapegoat, Discarded Partner, Overlooked Employee)

Welcome to the *other* side of the narcissist's twisted coin—the Devalued Supply. If you've ever felt like you went from being a narcissist's favorite person to their biggest disappointment overnight, congratulations! You've been *demoted*.

Scapegoat: In narcissistic families, the Scapegoat is the designated punching bag. No matter what goes wrong, it's *their* fault. Golden Child forgot their homework? The Scapegoat should have reminded them. Narcissistic Parent is in a bad mood? The Scapegoat must have *done something* to deserve it. This role is designed to keep one person permanently blamed so the narcissist never has to take responsibility for anything.

Discarded Partner: Remember that *Idealized Partner* from earlier? Yeah, this is their next stop on the emotional rollercoaster. The moment the narcissist decides they're no longer fun, useful, or obedient enough, the devaluation begins. Criticism replaces compliments, affection turns into coldness, and everything they once loved about you is now "annoying." Eventually, they'll discard you altogether—or keep you around just enough to watch you suffer.

Overlooked Employee: The workplace version of this is the employee who was once praised but now can't do anything right. Maybe they got *too* confident, maybe they started setting boundaries, or maybe the narcissistic boss just got bored. Whatever the reason, they've gone from being a star to being treated like an inconvenience.

Being the Devalued Supply is emotionally *brutal* because you're left wondering what you *did* to cause the switch. But here's the truth: *You didn't do anything*. The narcissist just needs someone to tear down, and today, you're the lucky winner. Tomorrow? It'll be someone else. And the cycle continues.

The Narcissist as the Puppet Master

Now, let's talk about the real star of the show—the narcissist. They aren't just a player in this twisted game; they're the *game master*. They decide who is favored, who is devalued, and when it's time to switch things up. And they *love* watching people scramble to figure out where they stand.

Why? Because as long as people are desperate for their approval, they *win*. If the Favored Supply is working overtime to stay on their good side, the narcissist gets endless validation. If the Devalued Supply is falling apart, the narcissist gets an ego boost from knowing they have that kind of control over someone's emotions. And if both sides are competing? That's the jackpot. Nothing strokes a narcissist's ego like watching people *fight for their attention*.

This is why narcissists *never* let things stay peaceful for long. If the Favored Supply gets too comfortable, they'll start throwing in little jabs to knock them down a peg. If the Devalued Supply starts pulling away, they might breadcrumb them with just enough attention to keep them hooked. And if both roles start questioning the system? Time to introduce *a new player*—because what's a drama without a surprise guest?

At the end of the day, the narcissist's ultimate goal is *control*. Whether they're idolizing, devaluing, or playing the people in their life against each other, it all comes down to keeping the spotlight on *them*. And as long as you're caught up in their game, you're not questioning the one thing they fear the most:

Why are you even playing at all?

How Narcissists Use Triangulation to Manipulate

Chapter 4:
Romantic Triangulation

Romance—the magical land where two people commit to each other, build trust, and create a partnership based on love and mutual respect. That is, unless a narcissist is involved. Then, it's a competitive bloodsport where the goal is to keep their partner anxious, insecure, and *always* working for their approval.

Welcome to *Romantic Triangulation*, where love triangles aren't just accidental dramas—they're *intentional strategies*. Narcissists don't just want to be loved; they want to be *chased, admired, and fought over*. And if that means dragging in exes, flirting with new prospects, or making their partner feel like they could be replaced at *any moment*, well… that's just good relationship management, right?

Love Triangles and Emotional Affairs

For most people, love triangles are *unfortunate situations*. For narcissists, they're *essential power plays*. Whether it's a real or *imaginary* third party, the narcissist thrives on creating tension, jealousy, and just enough uncertainty to keep their partner in a permanent state of insecurity.

There are a few signature moves in the narcissist's love triangle playbook:

> **The "Just a Friend" Setup:** They bring someone into the mix—an old friend, a coworker, or a *totally harmless* social media admirer—and make sure their partner *notices* how close they are. They might say, "Oh, we just *connect* on such a deep level" or "They really understand me in ways no one else does." You know, just innocent things that *definitely* won't make their partner spiral into self-doubt.

> **Fuel:** Maybe it's a little too much eye contact with the barista. Maybe it's a "harmless" DM to an ex. Maybe it's excessive praise of someone else's attractiveness. Whatever the method, the narcissist ensures their partner feels *uncomfortable*, but not enough to actually call them out without seeming "jealous" or "crazy."

The Emotional Affair Play: This is when the narcissist *technically* isn't cheating (or at least they'll swear they aren't), but their emotional energy is clearly invested elsewhere. Long, secretive conversations. An emotional bond that excludes their partner. Subtle (or not-so-subtle) comparisons. And of course, the classic line: "You're overreacting, we're *just friends.*"

The goal? Keep their partner *unsure* of where they stand. Because as long as their partner is fighting to keep their attention, they don't have time to realize that this entire dynamic is completely *insane.*

Ex-Partners and Future Faking

A narcissist's past relationships are *never* fully over. Why? Because exes are *perfect* tools for triangulation. Nothing says "You'd better keep proving yourself" like the looming presence of a former partner who is *mysteriously still in the picture.*

Some classic narcissist ex-related tactics include:

Keeping the Ex on a Pedestal: They'll casually bring up how *amazing* their ex was. "You know, my ex *always* used to do this for me," or "My ex really *understood* me in a way most people don't." The unspoken message? *Try harder.*

Keeping the Ex on the Hook: Whether it's the occasional "just checking in" text or a full-blown friendship, the narcissist *never* truly lets go. They might claim they're "just being mature," but what they're really doing is keeping their ex as a backup plan.

The "My Ex is Obsessed With Me" Routine: Sometimes, the narcissist flips the script and tells their current partner that their ex just *won't* let them go. "They're always reaching out," they'll say, conveniently ignoring the fact that they're *encouraging it*. This sets up their partner to feel like they have to *compete* with a ghost from the past.

And then there's **future faking**, the narcissist's favorite way to keep their partner hooked. They'll dangle an idealized future just out of reach—marriage, kids, vacations, *finally* committing—whatever their partner desperately wants. Of course, none of it ever actually happens. But as long as their partner *believes* it might, they'll stick around and tolerate *just a little more* manipulation.

Making the Partner Feel Replaceable

This is the ultimate goal of romantic triangulation—to keep the partner constantly questioning their worth, their security in the relationship, and whether they are *good enough* to keep the narcissist's attention.

Some tried-and-true tactics include:

> **Comparisons, Comparisons, Comparisons:** "I wish you were more like so-and-so." "Did you see how amazing that person looks?" "You used to be so much more fun." Anything to make their partner feel like they are *one step away* from being replaced.

> **Hot and Cold Behavior:** One minute, they're showering their partner with affection. The next, they're distant, disinterested, and vaguely implying that *someone else* might appreciate them more. This back-and-forth keeps their partner in a constant state of anxiety.

> **The Threat of "Options":** Whether it's a flirtatious friendship, an old flame still lingering, or the narcissist *suddenly* becoming hyperactive on dating apps "just to see what's out there," they make it *very* clear: their partner *is not* irreplaceable.

This dynamic creates *exactly* what the narcissist wants—a partner who is so desperate to *keep them*, they'll tolerate things they normally *never* would. And that's the whole point. As long as their partner is *competing* for their love, they hold all the power.

The Final Act: Breaking the Spell

The reality is, the narcissist *needs* triangulation more than they need love. Love requires vulnerability, honesty, and commitment—three things they avoid like the plague. But control? *That* is their true goal. And as long as they can keep their partner in a cycle of jealousy, insecurity, and competition, they can maintain that control indefinitely.

The only way to win? *Stop playing the game.* The second their partner stops reacting, stops trying to prove their worth, and stops engaging in the competition, the narcissist loses their hold. And nothing terrifies a narcissist more than a supply who refuses to be controlled.

So, the real question is: *Are you fighting for love, or just fighting to be "chosen"?* Because if it's the latter, maybe it's time to walk away from the rigged competition.

Chapter 5:
Familial Triangulation

Family—the place where love and support are supposed to be unconditional. But for a narcissist? It's just another playground for control, chaos, and pitting people against each other for their own amusement. A healthy family nurtures, but a narcissistic family? It turns relationships into a never-ending Hunger Games, where there's always a "favorite" and a "failure," and nobody ever feels truly safe.

If you grew up in this kind of environment, congratulations! You've survived the emotional equivalent of a gladiator arena. Now, let's break down the three major ways narcissists turn family members into unwitting players in their twisted little game.

Parent-Child Triangulation (Golden Child vs. Scapegoat)

Nothing screams *emotional stability* like a parent who decides their children should be categorized into "winner" and "loser." And that's exactly what narcissistic parents do with their infamous *Golden Child vs. Scapegoat* dynamic.

> **The Golden Child:** This kid can do no wrong. They are the apple of the narcissistic parent's eye, the "success story," the one who gets praised and protected at all costs. But don't get too jealous— being the Golden Child is just another form of control. Their worth is conditional. The moment they fail to live up to expectations, they risk becoming...

> **The Scapegoat:** This child, on the other hand, can do *nothing* right. They are blamed for everything, criticized endlessly, and made to feel like they are the root of all family problems. Why? Because a narcissistic parent needs someone to project their own flaws onto, and the Scapegoat is the perfect target.

And just to keep things *interesting*, the roles can switch at any time. Today's Golden Child can be tomorrow's Scapegoat if they step out of line, and vice versa. This ensures that both children stay anxious, desperate for approval, and endlessly competing for scraps of validation.

Sibling Rivalry Fueled by Narcissistic Parents

Think sibling rivalry is just a natural part of growing up? Not in a narcissistic household! Here, competition between siblings isn't just *encouraged*—it's *engineered*.

Narcissistic parents pit their children against each other in ways that ensure they never form a united front. Why? Because an isolated, insecure child is easier to control. The strategies include:

> **Comparisons Galore:** "Why can't you be more like your brother?" "Your sister always makes me proud, but you..." (insert disappointed sigh). The message? *You will never be enough unless you outshine your sibling.*

> **Creating Jealousy:** Giving one child privileges while depriving the other, then pretending they're just being "fair." Classic move.

> **Rewriting History:** If the Golden Child ever does something wrong, it's *forgotten or excused*. If the Scapegoat does something right, it's *downplayed or ignored*. Over time, this warps both siblings' perceptions of each other—and themselves.

The result? The siblings resent each other instead of realizing that the *real* villain in this mess is the narcissistic parent pulling the strings. And that's exactly the point.

Extended Family Conflicts Instigated by a Narcissist

But why stop at immediate family when you can create *multi-generational* dysfunction? Narcissists love to stir up drama within extended families, ensuring that even Thanksgiving dinner feels like a reality TV showdown.

Their favorite tactics include:

> **Spreading Misinformation:** The narcissist tells different family members different versions of the same story, twisting facts to make themselves the victim while turning everyone else against each other.

> **Playing the Martyr:** "I've *done so much* for this family, and yet nobody appreciates me!" This not only earns them sympathy but also makes others feel guilty for not catering to them.

> **Triangulating Through Gossip:** They tell *you* that your cousin said something nasty about you, then tell your cousin *you* said something nasty about them. The result? You both hate each other while the narcissist watches the fallout with a smug grin.

By the time you figure out what's happening, half the family has stopped speaking to each other, and the narcissist is sitting at the center of it all, pretending they *just want peace*.

Chapter 6:
Workplace Triangulation

The workplace should be a place of professionalism, collaboration, and teamwork, right? Well… not if a narcissist is in charge. Suddenly, the office transforms into their personal *Game of Thrones*, where favoritism, manipulation, and backstabbing aren't just possibilities— they're daily requirements. Meetings feel like strategy sessions in a reality show, casual conversations are loaded with hidden agendas, and everyone is constantly wondering, *Who's the favorite today? Who's about to get thrown under the bus?*

If you've ever felt like your office is more toxic than productive, you're not imagining it. Narcissists thrive on triangulating employees, and they do it with the precision of a master puppeteer. Let's break down some of their classic strategies:

Playing Employees Against Each Other
A narcissistic boss lives for employee conflict. Why? Because if everyone is busy competing, backstabbing, or

questioning each other, nobody has time to notice that their so-called "leader" is actually a chaos architect.

Feeding Different Stories: One day, they tell you, "You're the best worker we have," and the next, your coworker hears, "Your performance is slipping—maybe try to keep up with [insert your name]." Instant rivalry, guaranteed drama, and endless self-doubt. Bonus: everyone becomes hyper-aware of every small accomplishment or mistake, providing free entertainment for the narcissist.

Pitting Team Members Against Each Other: Conflicting deadlines, overlapping tasks, or conveniently "forgotten" instructions are all part of the show. Employees scramble, clash, and ultimately police each other's performance while the narcissist sits back, popcorn in hand, enjoying the chaos they've orchestrated.

Blaming One Employee for Another's Mistakes: Accountability? Ha! That's for mortals. If something goes wrong, someone has to take the fall—and the narcissist ensures it's someone else. Bonus points if the targeted employee starts resenting their coworkers, because then everyone's attention is off the narcissist and onto each other.

Public Praise, Private Criticism: Don't forget the classic carrot-and-stick maneuver. One team member is lauded in a meeting for their "outstanding work," while another is privately critiqued for the exact same behavior. Result? Confusion, jealousy, and a healthy dose of paranoia—the perfect fuel for the narcissist's fire.

Creating "Allies" to Isolate Others: They'll find someone eager to win their approval and turn that person into a mini-enforcer, passing on subtle digs, sharing half-truths, and helping maintain the tension among the rest of the team. Suddenly, no one can trust anyone fully, and the narcissist remains untouchable at the center of it all.

In short, when a narcissist is at the helm, the office stops being about productivity and starts being about control. Employees become pawns, collaborators become competitors, and every achievement or mistake is fodder for the drama machine. The more chaos they create, the safer they feel, because as long as everyone is distracted by each other, their leadership—and their ego—goes unquestioned.

Favoritism as a Manipulation Tactic

Narcissistic bosses always have a golden employee—a shining star in their eyes, a "pet" worker who is lavished with praise, given special privileges, and most importantly, wielded like a tool to keep everyone else in line. This favorite isn't just lucky—they're part of the narcissist's carefully orchestrated office theater. Their role is multifaceted, and it's as devious as it is demoralizing for the rest of the team.

This "favorite" employee serves a few purposes:

1. **The golden employee makes everyone else feel inferior.** While they're being applauded for their brilliance, the rest of the staff can't help but think, *What do they have that I don't?* Suddenly, everyone is working overtime to earn a shred of approval that may never come. Productivity skyrockets—but not because of leadership; because of anxiety, envy, and the desperate need to secure a spot in the narcissist's fleeting favor.

2. **They create an illusion of fairness.** The boss can point to their chosen favorite and proclaim, "See? I reward good work!" Problem solved, right? Except the favoritism has nothing to do with actual performance. It's about loyalty, compliance, and being the right kind of sycophant. Meanwhile, everyone else is left wondering why their exceptional work seems invisible while the chosen one

receives the spotlight for... well, showing up the "right" way.

3. **They are a temporary distraction, a pawn in an ongoing game.** Eventually, even the pet will be discarded—replaced with someone new—ensuring that everyone else stays on edge, perpetually guessing who will rise or fall next. The golden employee today could be yesterday's scapegoat tomorrow, and that uncertainty keeps the rest of the team scrambling, distracted, and subtly policing each other. It's chaos disguised as opportunity, insecurity disguised as inspiration, and drama disguised as leadership.

FYI, the golden employee isn't a reward—they're a warning. They're living proof that compliance, charm, or timing can temporarily elevate someone in the narcissist's eyes, but nobody is safe, nobody is permanent, and everyone is just part of the performance. And while the rest of the office nervously adjusts their behavior, the narcissist sits back, popcorn in hand, enjoying the show they wrote, directed, and produced.

Using Competition to Maintain Control

One of the narcissist's greatest workplace strategies is making employees *compete for basic respect*. They thrive on creating an environment where workers:

- Constantly doubt their own worth

- Feel like they're never doing *enough*

- Fear being replaced at any moment

This might come in the form of:

> **Unclear promotion opportunities:** "If you just work a little *harder*, maybe you'll get that raise." (Spoiler: You won't.)

> **Shifting goalposts:** What was "excellent work" last week is suddenly "not quite there" this week—because keeping employees in a constant state of insecurity gives the narcissist power.

> **Fake camaraderie**: The boss might act friendly one day, then ice-cold the next. This ensures employees are always trying to *win back* their approval.

The result? A workplace where nobody trusts each other, burnout is sky-high, and the narcissist sits comfortably at the top, untouched by the chaos they created.

The Bottom Line

Whether it's at home or in the office, triangulation serves the same purpose: *keeping people unstable, insecure, and fighting for the narcissist's attention.* The only way to escape? *Stop playing the game.*

Because at the end of the day, the biggest insult to a narcissist isn't confrontation. It's *indifference*.

Chapter 7:
Social and Friendship Circles

Friendships—those beautiful, supportive relationships where people uplift and respect each other. Unless, of course, there's a narcissist involved. Then, friendships become a strategic battleground where alliances shift, trust crumbles, and somehow, everything always circles back to *them*.

Narcissists don't just *participate* in social circles—they *control* them. They want to be the all-knowing, all-powerful center of attention, deciding who gets close and who gets cast out. And they achieve this by turning friends into enemies, planting seeds of doubt, and making sure *nobody* feels secure in their relationships.

So, let's break down how these social masterminds manipulate friend groups into absolute chaos—one toxic trick at a time.

The Narcissist as the 'Connector' Who Divides and Conquers

The narcissist—the self-appointed *social architect* of every friend group. They love positioning themselves as the glue that holds everyone together. "Without *me*, this group would fall apart," they say. And to *ensure* that remains true, they do what they do best: manufacture division while pretending to be the peacemaker.

Their favorite tactics include:

> **Selective Information Sharing:** They'll tell one friend a *slightly altered* version of what another friend said, ensuring misunderstandings and tension.

> **Playing Therapist (With an Agenda):** "Oh, you and Sarah had a fight? You should totally talk to me about it *instead of her*." Now they hold all the power.

> **Fostering Dependence:** They make everyone feel like they're the *only* trustworthy friend, subtly alienating others in the process.

In short, they present themselves as the *ultimate confidant*, all while feeding drama behind the scenes. And because they're so "charming" and "concerned," nobody sees the destruction until it's too late.

Turning Friends Against Each Other

Healthy friends support each other. Narcissists? They make sure *nobody* trusts anyone. After all, a group that sticks together is a group that might *compare notes* and realize who the real problem is.

Some signature moves include:

> **The "Did You Hear What They Said About You?" Routine:** Even if no such conversation happened, the narcissist will *casually* drop hints about how a friend might not be as loyal as they seem.

> **Creating Jealousy:** They shower one friend with attention while ignoring another, ensuring resentment festers. Bonus points if they later switch it up and pretend they *have no idea* why anyone feels left out.

> **Sabotaging Reconciliations:** If two friends start to mend a broken bond, the narcissist swoops in with *"new information"* or subtle reminders of past betrayals, ensuring the rift remains.

Their ultimate goal? Keeping everyone *distracted* with interpersonal drama so that nobody realizes the narcissist is the one stirring the pot.

Using Smear Campaigns to Isolate and Control

If a narcissist feels like someone is pulling away, getting too independent, or—worst of all—*seeing through their BS*, it's time for the grand finale: the **Smear Campaign**.

The smear campaign is their way of turning *everyone* against their target, ensuring that person is isolated, discredited, and too drained to fight back. And the best part? The narcissist gets to play the *victim* the whole time.

Here's how they execute it:

>**Dropping "Casual" Warnings:** "I hate to say this, but I think Alex might be a little… toxic. Just be careful around them." Congratulations, Alex is now officially on thin ice with the group.

>**The Fake Concern Strategy:** "I'm really worried about Jamie. They've been acting so unstable lately…" Translation: *I need you to doubt everything Jamie says about me.*

>**Flat-Out Lies:** If all else fails, they'll make up outrageous stories to destroy someone's reputation. And since narcissists are *really* good at playing the victim, most people believe them.

The goal? Making sure their target has *nowhere* to turn. A narcissist doesn't just want people to like them—they want to be the *only* source of social validation. If that means leaving someone completely isolated, so be it.

The Bottom Line

Narcissists don't have friends. They have **pawns, puppets, and potential threats**. Friendships aren't about connection for them—they're about control. And if that means tearing relationships apart, spreading lies, and keeping people in a constant state of insecurity, well… that's just another day in their social empire.

So if you ever notice that a certain "friend" always seems to be at the center of drama, stirring the pot while pretending to be the voice of reason—trust your gut. Because in the world of a narcissist, you're only valuable as long as you're useful.

And the second you stop playing along? You become the next villain in *their* twisted story.

Breaking Free from Triangulation

Chapter 8:
Recognizing When You're Being Triangulated

So, you think you're in a healthy relationship, maybe with a friend, family member, or partner? But then something feels… off. You're left questioning if it's you, if *they* are playing games, or if you've accidentally stumbled into the middle of a triangulation scheme.

Don't worry, this chapter is going to make it crystal clear—because recognizing triangulation is the first step to breaking free from it. Narcissists are masters at making you feel like you're the problem. Spoiler alert: you're not. Let's explore the red flags, emotional responses, and the way you can figure out which "role" you've been assigned in the narcissist's little circus.

Red Flags and Emotional Reactions

Triangulation isn't subtle. It's designed to stir up confusion, jealousy, and anxiety in those it targets. It's not about finding harmony—no, it's about keeping you off-balance. So, what does triangulation *really* look like? Well, here are some pretty obvious signs that you're being caught in the narcissist's web of manipulation:

Inconsistency in Attention: One minute, you're the best thing since sliced bread, and the next, you're nothing. The narcissist vacillates between idealizing you and devaluing you, creating emotional whiplash.

Unsolicited Comparisons: You'll find out they're comparing you to someone else (whether it's a romantic partner, sibling, or colleague), and it's always framed as a competition. "Why can't you be more like [insert name here]?"

Playing Both Sides: You might overhear or be told about private conversations that you weren't a part of—specifically, how "concerned" the narcissist is about someone else's opinion of you. They often create "he said, she said" scenarios to fuel confusion and distrust.

So, how do you react when you're in the middle of this madness? Most likely, you feel:

Anxiety about whether you're loved, appreciated, or even understood.

Jealousy or resentment toward someone else who seems to have the narcissist's favor.

Frustration over how hard you try to please them, only to feel like nothing's ever enough.

If these emotions sound all too familiar, welcome to the world of triangulation. The narcissist has *masterfully* manipulated your feelings to maintain control.

How to Identify if You're the Favored or Devalued Supply

Are you the "Golden Child" or the "Scapegoat"? Are you the one basking in attention and adoration, or are you stuck in a never-ending cycle of guilt and criticism? In the world of triangulation, you're *always* playing a role—and it's crucial to identify which one.

Favored Supply (Golden Child): You're the recipient of endless praise, admiration, and affection. They talk about you to others like you're the best thing since Wi-Fi. You feel *special*, but hold up—this attention is fleeting. It's not about *you* being genuinely appreciated. It's about the narcissist keeping you under their thumb as a source of validation. You're the shiny trophy in their collection, but don't get too comfortable.

- Red flags: Over-the-top compliments, "You're perfect," constant reminders of how much they need you, and a persistent effort to isolate you from other sources of validation.

Devalued Supply (Scapegoat):

You can do nothing right. They criticize your every move, and if you disagree, suddenly, you're "the problem." Don't be fooled—this is all part of the game. The narcissist needs someone to tear down so they can feel better about themselves. But here's the twist: they can flip the script at any time. One minute you're the "failure," and the next, they're trying to woo you back into the fold by pretending to care.

- Red flags: Constant criticism, being ignored, feeling blamed for everything that goes wrong, and confusion about the inconsistency in their behavior toward you.

If you feel like you're stuck in this cycle, it's likely the narcissist is swinging you between these two poles—one minute adored, the next, neglected. And the worst part? You can't win, no matter how hard you try.

The Psychological Impact of Triangulation

So, what's the mental fallout of all this nonsense? Well, the narcissist may be playing games, but you're the one left with the emotional wreckage. Triangulation does a number on your self-esteem and your perception of reality. It's a mental trap designed to make you doubt everything, especially your own instincts.

Here's how triangulation impacts the psyche:

Self-Doubt and Insecurity: The constant shifting of attention and affection makes you question your worth. One moment you're "the best," the next, you're a failure. This emotional rollercoaster eats away at your confidence.

Lack of Trust: Since triangulation is all about manipulation, it becomes nearly impossible to trust others. If you're constantly being pitted against other people, you start questioning everyone's intentions—including your own.

Emotional Burnout: The psychological toll of being manipulated and jerked around is exhausting. The constant need for validation, the fear of being discarded, and the hope that things might improve leave you mentally drained. You'll find yourself walking on eggshells, trying to predict the next mood swing.

Isolation: Over time, you'll start to feel like everyone else is "in on it" while you're the only one left in the dark. This creates a deep sense of loneliness as you struggle to make sense of the chaos the narcissist has created.

The impact of triangulation can last long after the narcissist has moved on to the next target. It leaves scars that are tough to heal, and a lingering mistrust of anyone who might resemble the narcissist in any way. But don't worry—recognizing it is half the battle. Once you see the game being played, you can start taking steps to remove yourself from the cycle.

The Bottom Line

Being triangulated is like being stuck in an emotional maze where you're constantly trying to figure out *which way is up*. But now that you know what to look for—red flags, emotional reactions, and your assigned role in the narcissist's playbook—you're equipped to spot triangulation before it gets too deep.

The key? Trust yourself. The narcissist wants you to doubt your perception, but you can absolutely break free from their mind games.

Chapter 9:
Strategies to Disengage

Let's talk disengagement. The dream we all have when we realize we've been sucked into a narcissist's tangled web of manipulation. But don't worry, it's not too late to step off the emotional rollercoaster. This chapter is your ultimate guide to cutting the strings, taking back control, and saying a big "no thanks" to the narcissist's chaotic games. It won't be easy, but it will be worth it.

We're talking about the three crucial steps to disengage from triangulation: **setting boundaries, avoiding emotional reactions that feed the cycle, and strengthening your self-worth**. With these strategies in place, you'll start to feel like you've finally emerged from the fog. So let's break it down.

Setting Boundaries and Refusing to Play the Game

Boundaries: a simple concept that narcissists *absolutely cannot stand*—because they thrive on bending others to their will. But here's the thing: once you set clear, non-negotiable boundaries, you stop being a puppet and become a person with agency.

Be Direct and Firm: When the narcissist tries to drag you into their triangle, **don't engage**. If they start talking about someone else in a way that feels manipulative, shut it down immediately with a calm, "I'm not going to discuss [person] with you," or "I don't want to be part of this conversation." No, you don't need to explain yourself. Just say no.

Consistent Enforcement: Setting a boundary once isn't enough. Narcissists will test your limits endlessly, so you need to repeat and reinforce your boundaries consistently. The more you let them slide, the more they will push. When they cross the line, don't hesitate to call it out. "We agreed I wouldn't be part of this, and you're still bringing it up. Please stop."

Limit Your Exposure: One of the easiest ways to disengage from the game is to *minimize your contact* with the narcissist. If they love playing the triangulation game over text or on the phone, step away. If it's happening in person, walk away. You have every right to protect your peace by removing yourself from the situation.

Once you stop playing their game, they lose their power. And trust me, they'll try to test you. But the more you stand your ground, the harder it will be for them to manipulate you.

Avoiding Emotional Reactions That Fuel the Cycle

Here's a fun fact: narcissists thrive on your emotional responses. If they can get you to react—whether it's anger, confusion, jealousy, or even anxiety—they know they've got you. Triangulation feeds off emotional chaos. So, if you want to disengage, the key is **maintaining emotional control** and refusing to let them see how much they've rattled you.

> **Stay Calm and Detached:** If you find yourself in a conversation where the narcissist is trying to provoke a reaction, take a deep breath. Keep your responses short and neutral. Don't get sucked into a long back-and-forth or explain your feelings— narcissists don't care about your feelings. They care about winning the game.

> **Practice the "Gray Rock" Method:** This is an emotional detox strategy where you become as uninteresting as a rock. Don't show excitement, frustration, or fear—be as bland, neutral, and non-reactive as possible. The less you engage emotionally, the less power they have over you.

> **Don't Bite the Bait:** If the narcissist tries to make you feel jealous or insecure by comparing you to

someone else—oh, look, they've found a new competitor in their imaginary "approval Olympics"—don't take the bait. Keep your cool, sip your metaphorical tea, and refuse to engage in the contest they've invented. You don't have to jump through hoops, earn points, or prove your worth in their rigged games. The moment you stop reacting, the thrill disappears for them, and suddenly you're boring. Yes, boring! And nothing terrifies a narcissist more than a target who refuses to perform on demand. Before long, they'll be off hunting for someone else who still flinches at every whisper, compliment, or sideways glance.

Here's the beauty of it: when you stop feeding the drama, you start to regain control of your own emotional thermostat. You decide when to feel, how to respond, and which battles—even imaginary ones—are worth your attention. The narcissist's well-rehearsed tricks, their half-truths, and their "subtle" digs lose their power because you're no longer dancing to their tune. You're no longer the puppet with strings tied to every whim or insecurity they provoke.

And the best part? As you become less reactive, the narcissist will start to realize that their usual bag of tricks isn't working. They may try harder at first—because, of course, they hate being ignored—but eventually, even their theatrics fall flat. Your calm, composed detachment is like kryptonite to their manipulative little games. No more frantic scrambling to please or compete. No more emotional rollercoasters engineered to keep you off-balance. You're finally watching from the sidelines, and the puppet strings have been cut. You're free, untouchable, and—dare we say it—completely unentertaining to the master manipulator.

In short: don't bite the bait. Don't engage. Don't sweat their manufactured crises. Because the second you stop reacting, the narcissist's power evaporates, and for the first time in a long time, you are in charge.

Strengthening Self-Worth and Independent Thinking

Let's face it: narcissists are experts at making you doubt yourself. Whether it's by devaluing you or constantly pitting you against others, their goal is always the same: make you feel small and dependent on them. The best way to disengage from triangulation is to **reclaim your sense of self-worth** and trust your own judgment.

Rediscover Your Value: Take a step back and remind yourself of your strengths, accomplishments, and what makes you *you*. Narcissists will make you feel like you don't measure up, but you know better. Spend time with people who support and validate you, and engage in activities that help you feel good about yourself.

Rebuild Your Confidence: The more you trust your own abilities and worth, the less power the narcissist has to manipulate you. Work on building your self-esteem by setting achievable goals, acknowledging your successes, and practicing self-compassion.

Question the Narcissist's Narratives: It's easy to start believing the narcissist's version of events, especially if you've been involved in triangulation for a while. But their reality is warped. If you feel like you're being unfairly vilified or pushed aside, *trust your gut*. Learn to listen to your own voice and make decisions based on your values—not the narcissist's twisted version of the truth.

When you strengthen your sense of self-worth and start thinking independently, you break the hold the narcissist has on you. No longer will you be swayed by their manipulation, and no longer will you be confused about your place in their toxic game. The truth will be clearer:

You are worthy of love, respect, and autonomy, regardless of what the narcissist tries to make you believe.

The Bottom Line

Disengaging from triangulation is a process, and it's not going to be easy. But by setting boundaries, avoiding emotional reactions, and strengthening your self-worth, you'll slowly but surely take back control. The narcissist may try to play the game, but you won't be there to play anymore.

Remember: You don't have to be part of their toxicity. You are worthy of peace, clarity, and emotional freedom. So, take a deep breath, stand firm, and watch as the narcissist loses their grip on you.

Chapter 10:
Healing and Moving Forward

So, you've identified the narcissist's games, disengaged from the emotional manipulation, and set healthy boundaries. But now comes the next (and often most difficult) step: **healing**. Breaking free from narcissistic triangulation and the toxic cycle of manipulation is a victory, but it's only the beginning of your journey to reclaim your life. In this chapter, we're going to focus on how you can rebuild trust in yourself and others, cultivate healthy relationships free from manipulation, and spot the warning signs of narcissistic dynamics in the future.

Let's take a deep breath—because healing is possible, and it starts with you.

Rebuilding Trust in Yourself and Others

After experiencing the mental and emotional chaos caused by narcissistic abuse, it's natural to feel a little… shaken. You may have been manipulated so thoroughly that trusting yourself feels impossible. But trust *can* be rebuilt. And the first place to start is with yourself.

Trust Your Instincts: Narcissists are experts at convincing you to doubt your gut. After all, when you're constantly told your perceptions are wrong, it can be hard to know when to trust yourself. But now that you're on the other side of the manipulation, listen to your instincts. Start small—when something doesn't feel right, acknowledge it. Your feelings are valid, and the more you trust your internal compass, the stronger your self-assurance will become.

Small Wins, Big Results: The more you act in alignment with your values and instincts, the more you'll see that your judgments are correct. Take time to reflect on past situations where you let doubt cloud your decisions, and begin making choices that align with your well-being and self-respect. With each success, your trust in yourself will grow.

Gradual Rebuilding of Trust with Others: After being betrayed and manipulated by a narcissist, trusting others may feel like an uphill battle. But remember, not everyone will treat you the way the narcissist did. Start with small interactions—look for honesty, consistency, and respect in others. Rebuilding trust with the right people takes time, but by setting boundaries and being cautious, you'll find relationships that are worth investing in.

It's going to take time to heal from the emotional scars left by the narcissist's manipulation, but the path forward is about reclaiming your agency and gradually restoring trust in yourself and others.

Cultivating Healthy Relationships Free from Manipulation

Now that you've broken free from the narcissist's toxic grip, it's time to focus on building new, healthier relationships that nourish you rather than drain you. Here's the thing: Healthy relationships aren't about perfection—they're about mutual respect, understanding, and support. So, how do you create these kinds of relationships?

> **Setting and Respecting Boundaries:** Healthy relationships require clear boundaries, and it's essential to communicate your needs and expectations. By practicing the same boundary-setting techniques you used to disengage from the narcissist, you'll ensure that your future relationships are built on mutual respect.

> **Trust, Communication, and Transparency:** Healthy relationships thrive on open and honest communication. Take time to express your needs

and listen to others. Foster an environment of respect where both parties feel valued and heard. Transparency is key, so never settle for relationships where you feel like you have to question someone's intentions or integrity.

Mutual Support and Understanding: The most fulfilling relationships are those where both parties are equally invested in each other's growth. Cultivate connections with people who celebrate your successes, offer support during tough times, and encourage your independence. A healthy relationship will not require manipulation or control—it will be an uplifting experience for both of you.

In these healthy, balanced relationships, you'll know your worth, and the people around you will know it too. And as you build these new connections, you'll be moving farther and farther away from the toxic patterns of narcissistic abuse.

How to Spot and Avoid Narcissistic Dynamics in the Future

Once you've healed from narcissistic abuse, the last thing you want is to get tangled up in those dynamics again. So, let's talk about how to spot red flags and avoid being sucked back into the narcissist's emotional web.

Watch for Love Bombing: Narcissists often reel you in with an intense, overwhelming display of affection and admiration in the early stages of a relationship. This is their way of securing their "supply," and it's important to be cautious if someone moves too quickly and floods you with attention. Healthy relationships build over time, not overnight.

Observe How They Handle Conflict: Narcissists avoid taking responsibility and are quick to shift blame. If someone seems to consistently avoid accountability or manipulates others into taking the fall, run the other way. Healthy people own their mistakes and communicate openly about problems.

Notice How They Treat Others: A narcissist will often devalue and disrespect people behind their backs while pretending to be kind to their face. Pay attention to how someone speaks about others, especially when those people aren't around. If they're constantly putting others down or spreading rumors, there's a good chance they're not someone you want to be close to.

Trust Your Instincts Again: Now that you've learned to trust yourself, trust your gut when something feels "off." If you feel manipulated, disregarded, or unsafe in a relationship, don't ignore those red flags. Walk away before you get too deep.

The more you pay attention to these signs, the easier it will be to spot and avoid narcissistic dynamics in the future. Healthy relationships are possible, but they require vigilance and self-awareness.

Conclusion of All Chapters

Triangulation and narcissistic abuse are insidious forces that chip away at your sense of self, leaving you feeling confused, insecure, and powerless. They thrive on your self-doubt, your need for validation, and your compassion—but here's the truth: none of it defines you. You've made it this far, and that is something to celebrate. You've recognized the manipulation, learned to see the patterns, and taken the first steps toward reclaiming your life. Each small step you take is a victory, a deliberate move away from the narcissist's control and toward your own freedom. You do not have to play the narcissist's game. You have the power to set boundaries, disengage, and heal. You are not responsible for someone else's chaos, nor are you obligated to endure manipulation to earn love or attention. Reclaiming your life may not happen overnight, but it is entirely within your reach. Every act of self-care, every boundary you enforce, every moment you refuse to comply with toxic expectations is a declaration of your strength.

To help you stay grounded, affirmations can be a powerful tool: I am worthy of love, respect, and genuine connection. I have the right to set boundaries and protect my peace. I trust myself to recognize manipulation and step away from it. I release the need to prove my worth to anyone who thrives on control. Each day, I grow stronger, wiser, and more in tune with my true self.

To anyone who still feels trapped in the cycle of narcissistic manipulation: You are not alone. You are resilient, capable, and deserving of kindness and respect. Healing is not a straight line—it comes with setbacks, moments of doubt, and emotional turbulence—but it is also a journey of immense growth, self-discovery, and empowerment. Celebrate every step forward, no matter how small, and recognize that progress is happening even when it doesn't feel immediate. The road to recovery can be rocky, but each step you take moves you closer to clarity, freedom, and peace. You are learning to reclaim your narrative, rebuild relationships that honor your boundaries, and trust in your instincts again. You are stronger than the manipulation, braver than the fear, and more capable than the cycle of abuse ever allowed you to believe. Believe in yourself, protect your heart, stand firm in your boundaries, and remember: the puppet strings have been cut, the master can no longer manipulate you, and your life is yours to reclaim. No more competing. No more complying. You have the victory. Game over. You've won.

Resources for Further Support

Healing from narcissistic abuse is a journey best traveled with support. If you need help along the way, there are many resources available to assist you:

- **Therapists specializing in narcissistic abuse recovery**

- **Support groups (online and in-person)**

- **Books on trauma recovery and self-empowerment**

- **Hotlines and crisis intervention services**

- **Online forums and communities for survivors of narcissistic abuse**

Don't hesitate to seek help, whether it's professional or from a trusted support system. You don't have to do this alone.

Interactive Journal: Reflecting on Narcissistic Triangulation and Healing

Welcome to your interactive journal, a space for you to reflect on what you've learned throughout this journey. This journal is designed to guide you through the concepts in each chapter and help you apply the insights to your life. The questions and activities are meant to promote self-awareness, healing, and clarity. Take your time with each section, and allow yourself the grace to process at your own pace.

Chapter 1:
What Is Triangulation?

Reflective Prompts:

1. **Understanding Triangulation**

   o How do you define triangulation based on your experience?

   o Have you witnessed triangulation in your relationships, whether romantic, familial, or at work? Describe the situations.

2. **Personal Experience**

   o How has triangulation affected your sense of self and your relationships with others?

   o Were there specific instances where you felt manipulated by being pitted against someone else?

3. **Shifting the Dynamic**

   o What was your initial emotional response when you discovered triangulation was happening to you?

   o How do you feel now, knowing that triangulation is a tactic used by narcissists?

Activity: Draw a diagram of a triangulation situation you've experienced. Who were the parties involved, and what roles did they play? How did it make you feel in that moment?

_____

_____

_____

_____

_____

_____

_____

_____

_____

_____

_____

_____

_____

_____

_____

_____

_____

_____

_____

_____

Chapter 2:
The Narcissistic Supply Chain

Reflective Prompts:

1. **Understanding Narcissistic Supply**

   o How would you describe the narcissistic supply in your life?

   o Were you aware that you were acting as a supply for a narcissist? How did that feel?

2. **Primary vs. Secondary Supply**

   o Reflect on the relationships where you may have been either a primary or secondary supply. What made you feel like you were valued or devalued?

3. **The Need for Multiple Sources**

   o Why do you think narcissists need multiple sources of supply? How does this affect the people in their lives?

Activity: Write a letter to your past self, expressing what you wish you had known about narcissistic supply and how you can reclaim your emotional independence going forward.

Chapter 3:
The Three Roles in Triangulation

Reflective Prompts:

1. **The Favored Supply**

   o Have you ever been in the "Golden Child" role? How did it feel to be idealized? How did the narcissist's attention impact your self-worth?

2. **The Devalued Supply**

   o Have you experienced being in the "Scapegoat" position? How did it affect your sense of identity and confidence?

   o Reflect on how it felt when the narcissist started to ignore, criticize, or belittle you.

3. **The Narcissist as Puppet Master**

   o What patterns did you notice when the narcissist pulled the strings? Did you ever feel like you were part of a larger manipulation scheme?

Activity: Write about a specific situation where you were either the favored or devalued supply. What emotional impact did it have on you? How did you react?

Chapter 4:
Romantic Triangulation

Reflective Prompts:

1. **Love Triangles and Emotional Affairs**

   o Have you ever found yourself in a love triangle? How did it feel to be caught in that dynamic?

   o Were emotional affairs involved? Reflect on how this altered your perception of trust and love.

2. **Ex-Partners and Future Faking**

   o Reflect on any instances where the narcissist made promises about the future that were never fulfilled. How did this affect your expectations and beliefs?

3. **Making the Partner Feel Replaceable**

   o Did you ever feel that you were replaceable or disposable in a romantic relationship? How did this affect your sense of worth?

Activity: Journal about any romantic experiences where triangulation occurred. How did you handle it, and what would you do differently today?

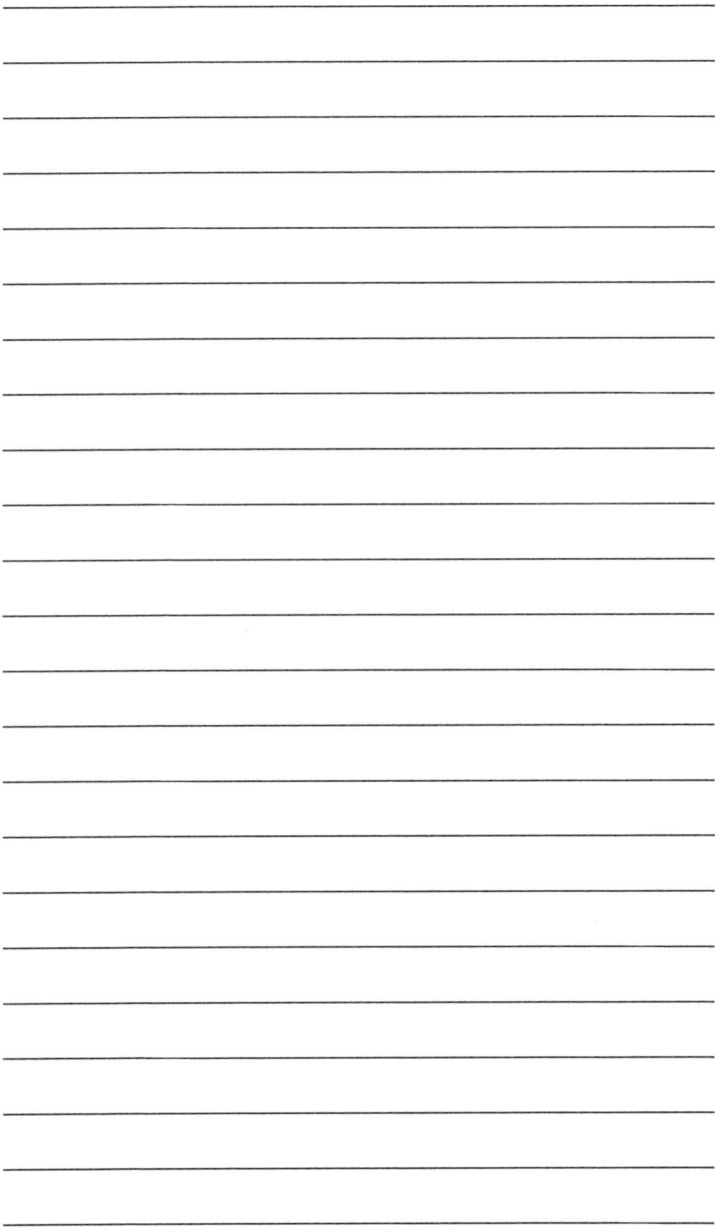

Chapter 5:
Familial Triangulation

Reflective Prompts:

1. **Parent-Child Triangulation**

   o How did your narcissistic parent's behaviors affect your family dynamic? Were you ever placed in the role of "Golden Child" or "Scapegoat"?

2. **Sibling Rivalry**

   o Reflect on how narcissistic dynamics affected your relationships with siblings. Were you encouraged to compete with each other?

3. **Extended Family Conflicts**

   o Did the narcissist play games with extended family? How did their actions cause division or confusion in family relationships?

Activity: Create a family tree or diagram showing the different roles within your family dynamic. Identify how triangulation may have influenced each relationship.

Chapter 6:
Workplace Triangulation

Reflective Prompts:

1. **Playing Employees Against Each Other**

    ○ Reflect on any workplace situations where a narcissistic boss or colleague played people against each other. How did this impact team morale and your sense of trust in others?

2. **Favoritism as Manipulation**

    ○ Did you ever feel like you were being "favored" in a way that wasn't genuine? How did this contribute to unhealthy competition?

3. **Using Competition to Maintain Control**

    ○ How did workplace competition affect your interactions with others? Did the narcissist thrive by causing division or manipulation?

Activity: Write about a time in the workplace where triangulation affected your work relationships. How did it impact your job satisfaction and well-being?

Chapter 7:
Social and Friendship Circles

Reflective Prompts:

1. **The Narcissist as the 'Connector'**

   o Reflect on any friendships where the narcissist tried to act as the "connector" between you and others. How did this dynamic impact your friendships?

2. **Turning Friends Against Each Other**

   o Did the narcissist attempt to turn you against a friend or manipulate you into competition with someone else? How did this affect your sense of loyalty and trust?

3. **Smear Campaigns and Isolation**

   o Reflect on any instances where the narcissist spread lies about you or tried to isolate you from your social circles. How did this impact your relationships?

Activity: Write a letter to a friend you've lost due to narcissistic triangulation, expressing how you feel about the situation and how you're moving forward.

Chapter 8:
Recognizing When You're Being Triangulated

Reflective Prompts:

1. **Red Flags and Emotional Reactions**

   o What were some emotional red flags you ignored when triangulation was happening?

   o How did those emotional reactions feel at the time, and how do you feel now about them?

2. **Identifying Your Role (Favored or Devalued Supply)**

   o Did you ever find yourself being cast as the "favored" or "devalued" supply? How did it shape your self-esteem?

3. **Psychological Impact of Triangulation**

   o How did being triangulated affect your mental and emotional health? Reflect on the lasting effects of these experiences.

Activity: Create a checklist of the red flags you've learned to watch out for in future relationships. What are the behaviors or tactics that you now recognize as triangulation?

Chapter 9:
Strategies to Disengage

Reflective Prompts:

1. **Setting Boundaries**

   o How do you currently approach setting boundaries in your relationships?

   o Reflect on any past relationships where you failed to set boundaries. What would you do differently now?

2. **Avoiding Emotional Reactions**

   o What techniques have you used to manage emotional reactions when the narcissist tries to provoke you? How has this helped you disengage from manipulation?

3. **Strengthening Self-Worth**

   o How do you nurture your self-worth and independence moving forward?

   o What are the steps you're taking to reclaim your confidence and sense of self?

Activity: Write a mantra or affirmation that reinforces your sense of self-worth and independence. Repeat this mantra daily as a reminder of your strength.

Chapter 10:
Healing and Moving Forward

Reflective Prompts:

1. **Rebuilding Trust in Yourself and Others**

   o   How are you rebuilding trust in yourself after narcissistic manipulation? What steps are you taking to trust others again?

2. **Cultivating Healthy Relationships**

   o   What does a healthy, nurturing relationship look like to you?

   o   How are you ensuring that your future relationships are free from manipulation?

3. **Spotting and Avoiding Narcissistic Dynamics**

   o   What are the key signs that you've learned to look out for in order to avoid narcissistic manipulation in future relationships?

Activity: Create a vision board or journal entry about your ideal healthy relationship. What qualities and values do you want to prioritize moving forward?

Conclusion

Congratulations on completing the interactive journal! By reflecting on these questions and activities, you've taken essential steps toward healing and reclaiming your personal power. Continue to journal regularly, as this can be a powerful tool in your journey to self-discovery and emotional recovery. Remember, healing is not linear—it's a process, but you are worthy of peace, joy, and authentic connection.

Works Cited

Bowen, M. (1978). *Family Therapy in Clinical Practice*. Jason Aronson.

The Bowen Center for the Study of the Family. (n.d.). Triangles. Retrieved from https://www.thebowencenter.org/triangles

Verywell Mind. (2019, September 16). What Is Triangulation in Psychology? Retrieved from https://www.verywellmind.com/what-is-triangulation-in-psychology-5120617

www.ingramcontent.com/pod-product-compliance
Lightning Source LLC
Chambersburg PA
CBHW052117030426
42335CB00025B/3025